Keto Diet Cookbook 2021

How To Lose Weight In 7 Days And Burn Fat Forever

Elena Harrison

Table of Contents

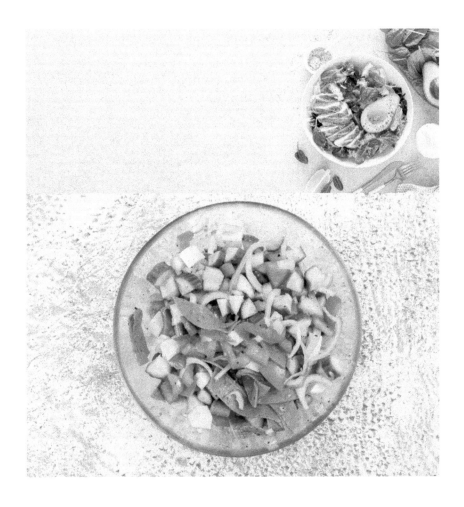

INTRODUCTION

The ketogenic diet has been highly praised and praised for the benefits of weight loss. This high-fat, low-carb diet has been shown to be extremely healthy overall. It really makes your body burn fat, like a talking machine. Public figures appreciate it too. But the question is, how does ketosis enhance weight loss? The following is a detailed picture of the ketosis and weight loss process.

Some people consider ketosis to be abnormal. Although it has been approved by many nutritionists and doctors. many people still disapprove of it. The misconceptions are due to the myths that have spread around the ketogenic diet.

Once your body is out of glucose, it automatically depends on stored fat. It is also important to understand that carbohydrates produce glucose and once you start a low carbohydrate diet, you will also be able to lower your glucose levels. Then your body will produce fuel through fat, instead of carbohydrates, that is, glucose.

The process of accumulating fat through fat is known as ketosis, and once your body enters this state, it becomes extremely effective at burning unwanted fat. Also, since glucose levels are low during the ketogenic diet, your body achieves many other health benefits.

A ketogenic diet is not only beneficial for weight loss, but it also helps improve your overall health in a positive way. Unlike all other diet plans, which focus on reducing calorie intake, ketogenic focuses on putting your body in a natural metabolic state, that is, ketosis. The only factor that makes this diet questionable is that this nature of metabolism is not very well thought out. By getting tattoos on your body regularly, your body will quickly burn stored fat, leading to great weight loss.

Now the question arises. How does ketosis affect the human body?

However, this phase does not last more than 2-3 days. This is the time it takes for the human body to enter the ketosis phase. Once you get in, you won't have any side effects.

You should also start gradually reducing your calorie and carbohydrate intake. The most common mistake dietitians make is that they tend to start eliminating everything from their diet at the same time. This is where the problem arises. The human body will react extremely negatively when you limit everything at once. You must start gradually. Read this guide to learn more about how to approach the ketogenic diet after 50.

Most fats are good and essential for our health so there are essential fatty acids and essential amino acids (proteins). Fat is the most efficient form of energy, and each gram contains about 9 calories. This more than doubles the amount of carbohydrates and protein (both have 4 calories per gram).

When you eat a lot of fat and protein and significantly reduce carbohydrates, your body adjusts and converts the fat and protein, as well as the fat that it has stored, into ketones or ketones, for energy. This metabolic process is called ketosis. This is where the ketogen in the ketogenic diet comes from.

BREAKFAST

1. Keto Omelet with Mushrooms

Preparation Time: 5 minutes

Cooking Time: 10 minutes

Servings: 1

Ingredients:

- 3 eggs
- 30 g butter for frying
- 30 g (60 ml) grated cheese
- 1/5 onion
- 3 pcs. mushrooms
- salt and pepper

Directions:

1. Break the eggs then put the contents into a small bowl.
2. Add salt and pepper to taste.
3. Beat the eggs with a fork until a uniform foam is formed.
4. In a pan, heat a piece of butter, and as soon as the butter has melted, pour the egg mixture into the pan.
5. When the mixture begins to harden and fry, and the eggs on top will still be liquid, sprinkle them with cheese, mushrooms, and onions (to taste).
6. Take a spatula and gently pry the edges of the omelet on one side, and then fold the omelet in half. As soon as the dish

begins to take a golden brownish tint, remove the pan from the stove then place the omelet on a plate.

Nutrition: Carbohydrates: 5 g Fats: 44 g Proteins: 26 g Kcal: 649

2. Cacao Crunch Cereal

Preparation Time: 5 minutes

Cooking Time: 0 minutes

Servings: 2

Ingredients:

- ½ cup slivered almonds
- 2 tablespoons coconut, shredded or flakes
- 2 tablespoons chia seeds
- 2 tablespoons cacao nibs
- 2 tablespoons sunflower seeds
- Unsweetened nondairy milk of choice (I use macadamia milk), for serving

Directions:

1. In a small bowl, mix the almonds, coconut, chia seeds, cacao nibs, and sunflower seeds. Divide between two bowls.
2. Pour in the nondairy milk and serve.

Nutrition: Calories: 325 Total Fat: 27 Protein: 10g Total Carbs: 17g Fiber: 12g Net Carbs: 5g

3. <u>Creamy Protein Muffins</u>

Preparation time: 5 minutes

Cooking time: 25 minutes

Servings: 12

Ingredients:

- 8 eggs

- 8 ounces cream cheese

- 2 tbsp whey protein

- 4 tbsp melted butter, cooled

Directions:

1. Heat up the oven to 350F.
2. Add melted butter and cream cheese in a bowl and mix.
3. Add whey protein and eggs into the bowl and mix until fully combined, using a hand mixer.
4. Put batter into a prepared muffin tin and transfer into the preheated oven.
5. Bake for 25 minutes.
6. Serve.

Nutrition: Calories: 165.1 Fat: 13.6g Carb: 1.5g Protein: 9.6g

KETO BREAD

4. Toast Bread

Preparation time: 3 1/2 hours

Cooking time: 3 1/2 hours

Servings: 8

Ingredients:

- 1 1/2 teaspoons yeast
- 3 cups almond flour
- 2 tablespoons sugar
- 1 teaspoon salt
- 1 1/2 tablespoon butter
- 1 cup water

Directions

1. Pour water into the bowl; add salt, sugar, soft butter, flour, and yeast.
2. I add dried tomatoes and paprika.
3. Put it on the basic program.
4. The crust can be light or medium.

Nutrition: Carbohydrates 5 g Fats 2.7 g Protein 5.2 g Calories 203 Fiber 1 g

5. <u>Low-Carb Cauliflower Bread</u>

Preparation Time: 20 minutes

Cooking Time: 45 min

Serving: 8

Ingredients:

- 2 cups almond flour
- 5 eggs
- 1/4 cup psyllium husk
- 1 cup cauliflower rice

Directions

1. Preheat broiler to 350 F.
2. Line a portion skillet with material paper or coconut oil cooking shower. Put in a safe spot.
3. In an enormous bowl or nourishment processor, blend the almond flour and psyllium husk.
4. Beat in the eggs on high for as long as two minutes.
5. Blend in the cauliflower rice and mix well.
6. Empty the cauliflower blend into the portion skillet.
7. Heat for as long as 55 minutes.

Nutrition: 398 Calories; 21g Fat; 4.7g Carbs; 4.2g Protein; 0

6. <u>Rosemary & Garlic Coconut Flour Bread</u>

Preparation Time: 20 minutes

Cooking Time: 45 min

Ingredients:

- 1/2 cup Coconut flour
- 1 sticks margarine (8 tbsp.)
- 6 enormous eggs
- 1 tsp. heating powder
- 2 tsp. Dried Rosemary
- 1/2-1 tsp. garlic powder
- 1/2 tsp. Onion powder
- 1/4 tsp. Pink Himalayan Salt

Directions:

1. Join dry fixings (coconut flour, heating powder, onion, garlic, rosemary, and salt) in a bowl and put in a safe spot.
2. Add 6 eggs to a different bowl and beat with a hand blender until you get see rises at the top.
3. Soften the stick of margarine in the microwave and gradually add it to the eggs as you beat with the hand blender.
4. When wet and dry fixings are completely consolidated in isolated dishes, gradually add the dry fixings to the wet fixings as you blend in with the hand blender.
5. Oil an 8x4 portion dish and empty the blend into it equitably.
6. Heat at 350 for 40-50 minutes (time will change contingent upon your broiler).

7. Let it rest for 10 minutes before expelling from the container. Cut up and appreciate it with spread or toasted!

Nutrition: 398 Calories; 21g Fat; 4.7g Carbs; 4.2g Protein; 0Sugars .5g

7. <u>Best Keto Garlic Bread</u>

Preparation Time: 10

Cooking Time: 15

Servings: 4

Ingredients:

- Garlic and Herb Compound Butter:
- 1/2 cup mellowed unsalted margarine (113 g/4 oz.)
- 1/2 tsp. salt (I like pink Himalayan salt)
- 1/4 tsp. ground dark pepper
- 2 tbsp. additional virgin olive oil (30 ml)
- 4 cloves garlic, squashed
- 2 tbsp. naturally slashed parsley or 2 tsp. dried parsley
- Topping:
- 1/2 cup ground Parmesan cheddar (45 g/1.6 oz.)
- 2 tbsp. crisp parsley

Directions:

1. Set up the Keto sourdough rolls by following this formula (you can make 8 standard or 16 smaller than usual loaves). The Best Low-Carb Garlic Bread

2. Set up the garlic margarine (or some other seasoned spread). Ensure every one of the fixings has arrived at room temperature before blending them in a medium bowl. The Best Low-Carb Garlic Bread

3. Cut the prepared rolls down the middle and spread the enhanced margarine over every half (1-2 teaspoons for each piece). The Best Low-Carb Garlic Bread

4. Sprinkle with ground Parmesan and spot back in the stove to fresh up for a couple of more minutes. The Best Low-Carb Garlic Bread

5. At the point when done, expel from the stove. Alternatively, sprinkle with some olive oil and serve while still warm.

Nutrition: Calories 270, Fat 15, Fiber 3, Carbs 5, Protein 9

8. Low Carb Flax Bread

Preparation Time: 10 minutes

Cooking Time: 24 min

Serving: 8

Ingredients:

- 200 g ground flax seeds
- 1/2 cup psyllium husk powder
- 1 tablespoon heating powder
- 1 1/2 cups soy protein separate
- 1/4 cup granulated Stevia
- 2 teaspoons salt
- 7 enormous egg whites
- 1 enormous entire egg
- 3 tablespoons margarine
- 3/4 cup water

Directions:

1. Preheat broiler to 350 degrees F.
2. Mix phylum husk, heating powder, protein disengage, sugar, and salt together in a bowl.
3. In a different bowl, blend egg, egg whites, margarine, and water together.
4. Slowly add wet fixings to dry fixings and consolidate.
5. Grease your bread dish with spread or splash.
6. Add blend to bread dish

7. Bake 15-20 minutes until set.

Nutrition: Cal: 20, Carbs: 3.5 g, Fiber: 8.5 g, Fat: 13 g, Protein: 10g, Sugars: 5 g.

9. Low Carb Focaccia Bread

Preparation Time: 10 minutes

Cooking Time: 25 min

Serving: 12

Ingredients:

- 1 cup almond flour
- 1 cup flaxseed feast
- 7 enormous eggs
- 1/4 cup olive oil
- 1 1/2 tablespoons heating powder
- 2 teaspoons minced garlic
- 1 teaspoon salt
- 1 teaspoon rosemary
- 1 teaspoon red bean stew chips

Directions:

1. Preheat your broiler to 350F.
2. In a blending bowl, join all your dry fixings and blend well.
3. Start including your garlic and 2 eggs one after another, blending in with a hand blender to get a mixture sort of consistency.
4. Add your olive oil last, blending it well until everything is joined. The more aerated the hitter turns into, the more "cushy" your bread will turn into.
5. Put every one of your fixings into a lubed 9x9 heating dish, smooth out with a spatula.

6. Bake for 25 minutes.

7. Let cool for 10 minutes and expel from the lubed heating dish.

8. Cut into squares and cut the squares down the middle. Add whatever you'd prefer to the center!

Nutrition: Cal: 50, Carbs: 2.5 g, Fiber: 4.5 g, Fat: 8 g, Protein: 8g, Sugars: 3 g.

10. Lemon & Rosemary Low Carb Shortbread

Preparation Time: 5 minutes

Cooking Time: 20 min

Serving: 6

Ingredients:

- 6 tablespoons margarine
- 2 cups almond flour
- 1/3 cup granulated Splenda (or other granulated sugar)
- 1 tablespoon naturally ground lemon get-up-and-go
- 4 teaspoons crisp pressed lemon juice
- 1 teaspoon vanilla concentrate
- 2 teaspoons rosemary*
- 1/2 teaspoon preparing pop
- 1/2 teaspoon preparing powder

Directions:

1. In a huge blending bowl, measure out 2 cups of almond flour, 1/2 tsp. heating powder and 1/2 tsp. preparing pop. Include 1/3 cup Splenda, or other granulated sugar to the blend. Put in a safe spot.

2. Zest your lemon with a Microplane until you have 1 Tbsp. lemon get-up-and-go. Squeeze a large portion of the lemon to get 4tsp lemon juice.

3. In the microwave, liquefy 6 Tbsp. of margarine and afterward include 1 tsp. vanilla concentrate.

4. Transfer your almond flour and sugar to a little blending bowl. Put your spread, lemon get-up-and-go, lemon squeeze, and slashed rosemary into the now vacant huge blending bowl. Include your almond flour once more into the wet blend gradually, mixing as you go. Continue blending until all the almond flour is included back.

5. Wrap the mixture firmly in cling wrap.

6. Place the enveloped batter by the cooler for 30 minutes, or until hard.

7. Preheat your stove to 350F, evacuate your batter, and unwrap it.

8. Cut your batter in ~1/2" increases with a sharp blade. In the event that this blade isn't sharp, it will cause the batter to disintegrate. On the off chance that the mixture is as yet disintegrating, that implies it needs additional time in the cooler.

9. Grease a treat sheet with SALTED margarine and spot your treats onto it.

Nutrition: Cal: 100, Carbs: 2g Fiber: 4.5 g, Fat: 10 g, Protein: 2g, Sugars: 4 g.

11. Low-Carb Garlic & Herb Focaccia Bread

Preparation Time: 10 minutes

Cooking Time: 25 min

Serving: 7

Ingredients:

- 1 cup Almond Flour
- 1/4 cup Coconut Flour
- 1/2 teaspoon Xanthan Gum
- 1 teaspoon Garlic Powder
- 1 teaspoon Flaky Salt
- 1/2 teaspoon heating Soda
- 1/2 teaspoon heating Powder
- Wet Ingredients
- 2 eggs
- 1 teaspoon Lemon Juice
- 2 teaspoon Olive oil + 2 teaspoons of Olive Oil to sprinkle
- Top with Italian Seasoning and TONS of flaky salt!

Directions:

1. Heat broiler to 350 and line a preparing plate or 8-inch round dish with the material.
2. Whisk together the dry fixings ensuring there are no knots.
3. Beat the egg, lemon squeeze, and oil until joined.
4. Merge the wet and the dry together, working rapidly, and scoop the mixture into your dish.

5. Make sure not to blend the wet and dry until you are prepared to place the bread in the broiler on the grounds that the raising response starts once it is blended!!!

6. Bake secured for around 10 minutes. Sprinkle with Olive Oil heat for an extra 10-15 minutes revealing to dark-colored tenderly.

7. Top with increasingly flaky salt, olive oil (discretionary), a scramble of Italian flavoring and crisp basil. Let cool totally before cutting for an ideal surface!!

Nutrition: Cal: 80, Carbs: 1g Fiber: 8.5 g, Fat: 7 g, Protein: 8g, Sugars: 10 g.

12. Cauliflower Bread with Garlic & Herbs

Preparation Time: 9 minutes

Cooking Time: 26 min

Serving: 12

Ingredients:

- 3 cup Cauliflower ("riced" utilizing nourishment processor*)
- 10 enormous Egg (isolated)
- 1/4 teaspoon Cream of tartar (discretionary)
- 1 1/4 cup Coconut flour
- 1 1/2 teaspoon sans gluten heating powder
- 1 teaspoon Sea salt
- 6 teaspoon Butter (unsalted, estimated strong, at that point softened; can utilize ghee for sans dairy)
- 6 cloves Garlic (minced)
- 1 teaspoon Fresh rosemary (slashed)
- 1 teaspoon Fresh parsley (slashed)

Direction:

1. Preheat the broiler to 350 degrees F (177 degrees C). Line a 9x5 in (23x13 cm) portion skillet with material paper.

2. Steam the riced cauliflower. You can do this in the microwave (cooked for 3-4 minutes, shrouded in plastic) OR in a steamer bin over water on the stove (line with cheesecloth if the openings in the steamer container are too huge, and steam for a couple of moments). The two different ways, steam until the

cauliflower is delicate and delicate. Enable the cauliflower to sufficiently cool to deal with.

3. Meanwhile, utilize a hand blender to beat the egg whites and cream of tartar until solid pinnacles structure.

4. Place the coconut flour, preparing powder, ocean salt, egg yolks, dissolved margarine, garlic, and 1/4 of the whipped egg whites in a nourishment processor.

5. When the cauliflower has cooled enough to deal with, envelop it by kitchen towel and press a few times to discharge however much dampness as could reasonably be expected. (This is significant - the final product ought to be dry and bunch together.) Add the cauliflower to the nourishment processor. Procedure until all-around joined. (Blend will be thick and somewhat brittle.)

6. Add the rest of the egg whites to the nourishment processor. Overlay in only a bit, to make it simpler to process. Heartbeat a couple of times until simply consolidated. (Blend will be cushioned.) Fold in the hacked parsley and rosemary. (Don't over-blend to abstain from separating the egg whites excessively.)

7. Transfer the player into the lined heating skillet. Smooth the top and adjust somewhat. Whenever wanted, you can squeeze more herbs into the top (discretionary).

Nutrition: Cal: 70, Carbs: 2.5 g, Fiber: 4.5 g, Fat: 15 g, Protein: 4g, Sugars: 3 g.

13. Grain-Free Tortillas Bread

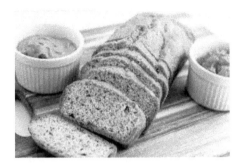

Preparation Time: 5 minutes

Cooking Time: 20 min

Serving: 5

Ingredients:

- 96 g almond flour
- 24 g coconut flour
- 2 teaspoons thickener
- 1 teaspoon heating powder
- 1/4 teaspoon fit salt
- 2 teaspoons apple juice vinegar
- 1 egg softly beaten
- 3 teaspoons water

Directions:

1. Add almond flour, coconut flour, thickener, preparing powder and salt to nourishment processor. Heartbeat until completely joined. Note: you can, on the other hand, whisk everything in

a huge bowl and utilize a hand or stand blender for the accompanying advances.

2. Pour in apple juice vinegar with the nourishment processor running. When it has dispersed equally, pour in the egg. Pursued by the water, stop the nourishment processor once the batter structures into a ball. The batter will be clingy to contact.

3. Wrap mixture in stick film and ply it through the plastic for a moment or two. Consider it somewhat like a pressure ball. Enable the mixture to rest for 10 minutes (and as long as three days in the refrigerator).

4. Heat up a skillet (ideally) or container over medium warmth. You can test the warmth by sprinkling a couple of water beads if the drops vanish promptly your dish are excessively hot. The beads should 'go' through the skillet.

5. Break the mixture into eight 1" balls (26g each). Turn out between two sheets of material or waxed paper with a moving pin or utilizing a tortilla press (simpler!) until each round is 5-crawls in distance across.

6. Transfer to skillet and cook over medium warmth for only 3-6 seconds (significant). Flip it over promptly (utilizing a meager spatula or blade), and keep on cooking until just daintily brilliant on each side (however with the customary roasted imprints), 30 to 40 seconds. The key isn't to overcook them, as they will never again be flexible or puff up.

7. Keep them warm enclosed by kitchen fabric until serving. To rewarm, heat quickly on the two sides, until simply warm (not exactly a moment)

Nutrition: Cal: 70, Carbs: 2.2g Fiber: 4.5 g, Fat: 8 g, Protein: 8g, Sugars: 3 g.

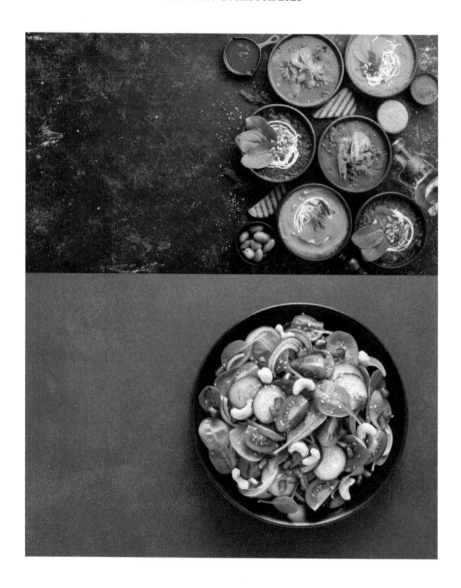

KETO PASTA

14. Creamy Zoodles

Preparation time: 2 minutes

Cooking time: 3 minutes

Servings: 1

Ingredients:

- Three (3) cloves of minced garlic
- Two (2) tablespoons of butter
- Two (2) medium zucchini
- A quarter teaspoon salt to taste
- A quarter teaspoon pepper
- A quarter cup of parmesan cheese

Directions:

1. Wash your zucchini then cut it to strands using a spiralizer or vegetable peeler then set aside. If done right, your zucchini should come out like spaghetti strands. I mean, that's the point right?

2. Put a large pan on medium heat. Put the butter in to melt and then add minced garlic. Stir fry the garlic until it starts to appear translucent. If you know you have an affinity for burning things, please be attentive so the garlic doesn't get burnt.

3. Add your zucchini strands and stir fry for three minutes. Make sure to taste your noodle strands to check how tender they are as zucchini cooks really fast. Try not to "taste" till it finishes.

4. Bring down the pan, add salt, pepper and parmesan cheese, stir until well combined and serve..

Nutrition: Calories: 100 Total Fat: 4g Carbs: 4g Protein: 4g

15.<u>Keto Carbonara Pasta</u>

Preparation time: 10 minutes

Cooking time: 15 minutes

Servings: 1

Ingredients:

- 150 grams of bacon
- One large egg yolk
- A packet of miracle noodles
- A cup of heavy whipping cream
- Two (2) tablespoons of parmesan cheese
- 60 grams of chicken breast

Directions:

1. Dice the chicken and Chicken in separate plates.
2. Set both to cook separately in a frying pan for 5 minutes.
3. Note: Do not let the bacon become crispy.
4. Put parmesan cheese and egg yolk in a small bowl and mix until it forms a paste.
5. Pour the cheese mixture into a frying pan and put on medium heat.
6. Add half the amount of cream and mix until a smooth creamy paste is formed.
7. Add the other half of the cream,bacon and chicken. Stir until fully coated.
8. Dry fry miracle noodles in another pan for 10 minutes, stirring continuously so it doesn't stick or burn.

9. Mix the noodles with sauce and serve.

Nutrition: Calories: 580 Total Fat: 50g Carbs: 5g Protein: 27g

16.Egg Pasta

Preparation time: 40 minutes

Cooking time: 25 minutes

Servings: 1

Ingredients

- One large egg yolk
- A cup of low moisture Mozzarella cheese (shredded)

Directions

1. Put the mozzarella into a point and microwave for 1-2 minutes
2. Take the cheese out and stir until fully melted. If cheese appears to have lumps, microwave for 1 more minute.
3. Let cool for 1-3 minutes before adding the egg (to avoid scrambling it).
4. Stir the yolk and cheese mixture until you have a smooth yellow dough.
5. Line a flat surface with a piece of parchment paper and place your dough on it.
6. Cover the dough with another parchment and use a rolling pin to flatten and thin out. Continue thinning it out until your dough is less than a quarter inch thick.
7. Remove the top parchment and cut your dough into long, thin strips.
8. When you are done,place your strips of dough (with bottom piece of parchment paper) on a flat tray or plate and put into the refrigerator to dry out.

9. Put in the pasta and let cook for 1 minute. You have to be careful not to overcook if or the pasta will begin to break and melt.

10. Once the pasta is ready, sieve and run under cold water to cool.

11. Use your hands to gently peel apart any strands that might be glued together.

Nutrition: Calories: 358 Total Fat: 22g Carbs: 3g Protein: 33g

17.Palmini Low-Carb Pasta

Preparation time: 5 minutes

Cooking time: 2 minutes

Servings: 1

Ingredients:

- A tablespoon of butter
- Two (2) tablespoons of parmesan cheese (shredded)
- Four (4) fresh basil leaves
- A quarter teaspoon of black pepper.
- A can of palmini linguine (drained and rinsed)
- A quarter teaspoon of salt

Directions:

1. Boil the drained and rinsed palmini in a pot of water for five minutes on medium heat.
2. Drain the palmini.
3. Put the cheese and butter in a bowl and microwave for 1 minute or until fully melted.
4. Sprinkle some salt on the parmini and pour it into the melted cheese, add pepper and serve with a few leaves of fresh basil.

Nutrition: Calories: 201 Total Fat: 14g Carbs: 12g Protein: 9g

18. Keto Shirataki Noodles

Preparation time: 2 minutes

Cooking time: 3 minutes

Servings: 1

Ingredients:

- A tablespoon of unsalted butter
- A quarter cup of grated Parmesan
- A quarter teaspoon of garlic powder
- A quarter teaspoon of Kosher salt
- A quarter teaspoon of black Pepper
- A pack of miracle noodles

Directions:

1. Drain and rinse noodles because they tend to have a fishy smell.
2. Put a large pan on medium-low and dry-roast the noodles.
3. Add butter, salt, garlic powder, and pepper. Stir fry.
4. Turn off the heat and put the noodles into a plate.
5. Sprinkle some parmesan cheese and serve.

Nutrition: Calories: 0 Total Fat: 0g Carbs: 0g Protein: 0g

19.Keto Butter Cabbage Noodles

Preparation time: 5 minutes

Cooking time: 10 minutes

Servings: 2

Ingredients:

- A quarter cup of unsalted butter
- A teaspoon of dried oregano
- A clove of garlic (diced)
- Half a cup of parmesan cheese (shredded)
- A teaspoon of salt
- A teaspoon of dried basil
- A head of green cabbage
- A quarter cup of red pepper flakes
- Half a bulb of onion

Directions:

1. Wash the cabbage and cut into thin long strips then set aside.
2. Dice the onion and garlic then set aside
3. Melt butter on medium -high in a non-stick frying pan
4. Saute the minced onion and garlic until they start to brown.
5. Add chili flakes, salt and herbs and stir until well combined.
6. Add the cabbage and stir until it is fully coated in the mixture.
7. Cook for 2-3 minutes or until it loses moisture and starts to wilt.
8. Note: If you cook it for too long, it will lose too much moisture and become too soft. We want it to have a spaghetti

feel to it, so turn it down when it can perfectly fold around a fork.

9. Put the cabbage in a plate and sprinkle some parmesan cheese on top then serve.

10. You can spice up your cabbage noodles with some diced chicken, bacon or minced beef.

Nutrition: Calories: 187 Total Fat: 5g Carbs: 1g Protein: 3g

20. Keto Shrimp Scampi

Preparation time: 20 minutes

Cooking time: 10 minutes

Servings: 1

Ingredients:

- A quarter cup of chicken broth
- A quarter teaspoon of red chili flakes
- A pinch of salt
- One pound of shrimp
- A clove of garlic (minced)
- Two (2) tablespoons of parsley (chopped)
- Two (2) tablespoons of lemon juice
- Two (2) tablespoons of unsalted butter
- Two (2) summer squash

Directions:

1. Slice the squash.
2. Sprinkle with salt and spread the noodles on an absorbent piece of parchment or paper towel, set aside for 15 minutes.
3. Use the paper towel to wring out the excess moisture in the noodles.
4. In a non-stick pan, melt butter, and stir fry garlic until it starts to turn brown.
5. Add lemon juice, chicken broth and chili flakes, stir and set on medium-low for 3 minutes.

6. Merge the shrimp, let boil for another 3 minutes or until shrimps start to turn a light shade of pink, then reduce the heat to low and let it simmer.

7. Taste the sauce and add pepper and salt to your liking.

8. Put in the summer squash noodles and parsley, stirring gently so as to coat the noodles in the sauce.

Nutrition: Calories: 334 Total Fat: 13.1g Carbs: 2.49g Protein: 48.4g

21.<u>Vietnamese Pasta Bowl</u>

Preparation time: 20 minutes

Cooking time: 25 minutes

Servings: 1

Ingredients:

- A pinch of salt
- A quarter pounder of shrimp Butterfield
- 25 grams of chopped peanuts
- Half a cup of cucumber
- Four(4) cups of romaine's lettuces (chopped)
- 25 great of pork ribs(thinly cut)
- Two (2) packs of Shirataki noodles (rinsed and drained)
- Nine (9) sprigs of cilantro
- 20 grams of sprouted mung beans
- A pound of boneless country style
- A quarter cup of fish sauce (Red coat)
- Two (2) tablespoons of white rice vinegar
- A quarter cup of water
- Two (2) tablespoons of Erythritol
- A tablespoon spoon of garlic chili sauce

Directions:

1. Boil the noodles for 3-5 minutes, then drain.
2. Put the noodles in the fridge until the salad is ready to be served.

3. Sprinkle some salt on shrimps and pork ribs and grill until well cooked, then set aside.

4. Share the already prepared sales ingredients into four different bowls.

5. Note: The bowls should be big enough to stir and toss salad in without spilling.

6. Put the cooked noodles, romaine, cooked shrimp and pork, cilantro, peanuts, cucumber and mung beans.

7. Put fish sauce, white rice vinegar, garlic chili sauce, Erythritol and water in a bowl and mix until well combined.

8. Drizzle a generous amount over your salad, then toss to combine. Serve as desired.

Nutrition: Calories: 300 Total Fat: 17g Carbs: 4g Protein: 31g

22.   <u>Keto Japanese Seafood Pasta</u>

Preparation time: 5 minutes

Cooking time: 10 minutes

Servings: 2

Ingredients:

- Two (2) cloves of garlic
- Three (3) tablespoons of Heavy cream
- Half an onion(diced)
- Half a cup of Clam juice
- A teaspoon of soy sauce
- A tablespoon of salted butter
- A pack of Shirataki noodles
- A quarter teaspoon of black pepper
- A tablespoon of Kewpie mayo
- Two (2) tablespoons of white wine
- Frozen seafood mix (preferably shrimp, clams and bay scallops)

Directions:

1. If your seafood mix is frozen, thaw it until fully melted.
2. Boil a water.
3. Strain the shirataki noodles to get rid of pre-packed liquid.
4. Run the noodles under cold water, put in a bowl then set aside.
5. Dice the onions and garlic then set aside.

6. Put soy sauce, kewpie mayo, and heavy cream into a small bowl then mix until fully combined then set aside.

7. Attach in the shirataki noodles, and cook for 2-3 minutes (this is mostly to remove the taste of the pre-packed liquid from the noodles)

8. Strain the noodles and set aside.

9. Fry onions until it starts to turn brown.

10. Add white wine, seafood mix, clam juice and garlic and cook, stirring until seafood gets completely cooked through and the liquid in the pan dries up.

11. Pour in the sauce from step 5 and reduce the heat to low. Stir the mixture until full combined and let cook for another minute.

12. Pour the sauce over the shirataki noodles and enjoy!

Nutrition: Calories: 325 Total Fat: 11g Carbs: 4g Protein: 14g

23. <u>Low carb Spaghetti & Fettuccine</u>

Preparation time: 2 minutes

Cooking time: 3 minutes

Servings: 1

Ingredients:

- Three (3) cloves of minced garlic
- Two (2) tablespoons of butter
- Two (2) medium zucchini
- A quarter teaspoon salt to taste
- A quarter teaspoon pepper
- A quarter cup of parmesan cheese

Directions:

1. Wash your zucchini then cut it to strands using a spiralizer or vegetable peeler then set aside. If done right, your zucchini should come out like spaghetti strands. I mean, that's the point right?

2. Put a large pan on medium heat. Put the butter in to melt and then add minced garlic. Stir fry the garlic until it starts to appear translucent. If you know you have an affinity for burning things, please be attentive so the garlic doesn't get burnt.

3. Add your zucchini strands and stir fry for three minutes. Make sure to taste your noodle strands to check how tender they are as zucchini cooks really fast. Try not to "taste" till it finishes.

4. Bring down the pan, add salt, pepper and parmesan cheese, stir until well combined and serve..

Nutrition: Calories: 100 Total Fat: 4g Carbs: 4g Protein: 4g

24. Tri-Color Bell Pepper Antipasto Salad With Olives And Tuna

Preparation time: 5 minutes

Cooking time: 10 minutes

Serves: 4

Ingredients:

- 2 (6-ounce) cans tuna, drained
- 1/2 cup sliced black olives
- 1/4 cup balsamic vinaigrette (see here)
- 1 green bell pepper, spiralized
- 1 yellow bell pepper, spiralized
- 1 red bell pepper, spiralized
- 1/2 cup cherry tomatoes, halved
- Salt
- Freshly ground black pepper

Directions:

1. In a large bowl, mix to combine the tuna and olives with the balsamic vinaigrette. Add the bell pepper noodles and cherry tomatoes and toss to combine. Season with salt and pepper and serve immediately.

Nutrition: Calories 270 Fat 15g, Protein 24g, Sodium 603mg, Carbs 1g, Fiber 2g

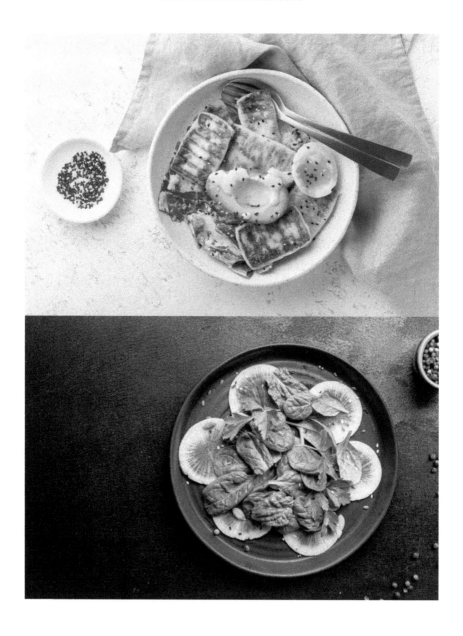

KETO CHAFFLE

25.   Coconut-Olive Chaffles

Preparation Time: 4 minutes

Cooking Time: 10 minutes

Servings: 2

Ingredients:

- Coconut flour – 1 teaspoon

- Eggs – 2

- Water – 2 tablespoons

- Olive oil – 2 tablespoons

- Garlic powder – 1/2 teaspoon

- Baking powder – 1/8 teaspoon

Directi:ons

1. Mix all ingredients in one bowl

2. Preheat waffle iron and lightly grease it

3. Pour mixture and spread evenly

4. Cook till crisp

5. Takes 10 min to prepare and serves 2

Nutrition: Calories 139 Total Fat 4.6 g Total Carbs 2.5 g Sugar 6.3 g
Fiber 0.6 g Protein 3.8 g

26.   Duckfila Chaffles

Preparation Time: 5 minutes

Cooking Time: 20 minutes

Servings: 2

Ingredients:

- Seared duck breast pieces – 1
- Pickle juice – 4 tablespoons
- Parmigiano cheese – 4 tablespoons
- Pork rinds – 2 tablespoons
- Butter – 1 teaspoon
- Flaxseed (ground) – 1 teaspoon
- Salt (as desired)
- Black pepper powder – 1/4 teaspoon
- For bun
- Shredded mozzarella – 1 cup
- Egg – 1
- Butter extract – 1/4 teaspoon
- Stevia glycerite – 4 drops

Directions:

1. Cut half- inch duck pieces and soak in pickle juice for one hour minimum
2. Pre-heat air fryer
3. Mix all other duck ingredients in one bowl
4. Drain pickle juice and add duck into bowl

5. Let duck cook for 6 min on each side at 400°

6. Mix all bun ingredients together in one bowl

7. Place in waffle maker to cook for about 4 min

8. Sandwich the cooked duck between the buns

Nutrition: Calories 139 Total Fat 4.6 g Total Carbs 2.5 g Sugar 6.3 g Fiber 0.6 g Protein 3.8 g

27. Bacon and Sour Cream Chaffles

Preparation Time: 5 minutes

Cooking Time: 20 minutes

Servings: 2

Ingredients:

- Cheddar – 1 cup
- Sour cream – 3 tablespoons
- American cheese – 2 slices
- Bacon pieces – 4
- Sour cream – 2 tablespoons

Directions:

1. Pre-heat and grease waffle maker
2. Mix Sour cream and cheddar cheese together
3. Pour mixture onto waffle plate and cook till crunchy
4. Cook bacon pieces till crispy then dry then
5. Fry Sour cream and add it in between two chaffles alongside bacon and cheese slices

Nutrition: Calories 115 Fat 7.3g Protein 1.4g Carbs: 4g

28.   Quinoa Parmigiano-Reggiano Chaffles

Preparation Time: 5 minutes

Cooking Time: 5 minutes

Servings: 2

Ingredients:

- Parmigiano-Reggiano cheese (shredded) – 1 cup
- Eggs – 2
- Quinoa flour – 2 tablespoons

Directions:

1. Pre-heat and grease waffle iron
2. Mix Parmigiano-Reggiano cheese and eggs in one bowl
3. Add the Quinoa flour into mixture to enhance texture
4. Pour mixture onto waffle plate and cook till crunchy
5. Garnish ready and slightly cooled chaffles with preferred garnish
6. Takes 5 min to prepare and serves 2

Nutrition: Calories 115 Fat 7.3g Protein 1.4g Carbs: 4g

29. Bacon Provolone Chaffles

Preparation Time: 5 minutes

Cooking Time: 15 minutes

Servings: 2

Ingredients:

- Provolone cheese (shredded) – 1 cup
- Eggs – 2
- Green onion (diced) – 1 tbsp
- Italian seasoning – 1/2 teaspoon
- Bacon – 4 strips
- Tomato (sliced) - 1
- (c) Butter head lettuce – 2 leaves
- Mayo – 2 tablespoons

Directions:

1. Pre-heat and grease waffle maker
2. Mix all ingredients in one bowl
3. Pour mixture onto waffle plate and spread evenly
4. Cook till crunchy then leave to cool for a minute
5. Serve with butter head lettuce, tomato and mayo

Nutrition: Calories 115 Fat 7.3g Protein 1.4g Carbs: 4g

30. **Chicken Chickpea Chaffles**

Preparation Time: 5 minutes

Cooking Time: 10 minutes

Servings: 2

Ingredients:

- Provolone cheese (shredded) – 1 cup
- Eggs – 2
- Butter head Lettuce (optional) – 2 leaves
- Ketchup (sugar free) – 2 tablespoons
- Soy sauce – 1 tablespoon
- Worcestershire/Worcester sauce – 2 tablespoons
- Monk fruit/swerve – 1 teaspoon
- Chicken thigh (boneless) – 2 pieces
- Chickpea flour – 3/4 cup
- Salt (as desired)
- Eggs – 1
- Black pepper – (as desired)
- Vegetable cooking oil – 2 cups
- Pork rinds – 3 oz
- Salt – 1 tablespoon
- Water – 2 cups

Directions:

1. Boil chicken for 30 min then pat it dry
2. Add black pepper and salt to the chicken

3. Mix soy sauce, Worcestershire sauce , ketchup and Swerve/Monkfruit in one bowl then set aside

4. Grind pork rinds into fine crumbs

5. In separate bowls, add the Chickpea flour, beaten eggs and the crushed pork then coat your chicken pieces using these ingredients in their listed order

6. Fry coated chicken till golden brown

7. Pre-heat and grease waffle maker

8. Mix eggs and Provolone cheese together in a bowl

9. Pour into waffle maker and cook till crunchy

10. Wash and dry green lettuces

11. Spread previously prepared sauces on one chaffle, place some lettuce, one chicken katsu then add one more chaffle

Nutrition: Calories: 125 Fat: 7g Carb: 1 g Protein: 5g

KETO BREAD MACHINE

31.Pita Bread

Preparation Time: 10 minutes

Cooking Time: 15 minutes

Servings: 8

Ingredients:

- 2 cups almond flour, sifted
- 1/2 cup water
- 2 Tbsp. olive oil
- Salt, to taste
- 1 tsp. black cumin

Directions:

1. Preheat the oven to 400F.
2. Combine the flour with salt. Add the water and olive oil.
3. Massage the dough and let stand for 15 minutes.
4. Shape the dough into 8 balls.
5. Put a parchment paper on the baking sheet and flatten the balls into 8 thin rounds.
6. Sprinkle black cumin.
7. Bake for 15 minutes, serve.

Nutrition: Calories: 73 Fat: 6.9g Carb: 1.6g Protein: 1.6g

32.   **Bread De Soul**

Preparation Time: 10 minutes

Cooking time: 45 minutes

Servings: 16

Ingredients:

- 1/4 tsp. cream of tartar
- 2 1/2 tsp. baking powder
- 1tsp. xanthan gum
- 1/3 tsp. baking soda
- 1/2 tsp. salt
- 2/3 cup unflavored whey protein
- 1/4 cup olive oil
- 1/4 cup heavy whipping cream
- 2drops of sweet leaf stevia
- 2egg
- 1/4 cup butter
- 12 oz. softened cream cheese

Directions:

1. Preheat the oven to 325F.
2. Using a bowl, microwave cream cheese and butter for 1 minute.
3. Remove and blend well with a hand mixer.
4. Add olive oil, eggs, heavy cream, and few drops of sweetener and blend well.
5. Blend the dry ingredients in another bowl.

6. Mix the wet ingredients with the dry ones and mix using a spoon. Don't use a hand blender to avoid whipping it too much.

7. Lubricate a bread pan and pour the mixture into the pan.

8. Bake in the oven until golden brown, about 45 minutes.

9. Cool and serve.

Nutrition: Calories: 200 Fat: 15.2g Carb: 1.8g Protein: 10g

MAINS

33.   Stuffed Chicken Breasts

Preparation time: 30 minutes

Cooking time: 30 minutes

Servings:4

Ingredients:

- tablespoon butter

- ¼ cup chopped sweet onion

- ½ cup goat cheese, at room temperature

- ¼ cup Kalamata olives, chopped

- ¼ cup chopped roasted red pepper

- tablespoons chopped fresh basil

- (5-ounce) chicken breasts, skin-on

- 2 tablespoons extra-virgin olive oil

Directions:

1. Preheat the oven to 400°F.

2. In a small skillet over medium heat, melt the butter and add the onion. Sauté until tender, about 3 minutes.

3. Transfer the onion to a medium bowl and add the cheese, olives, red pepper, and basil. Stir until well blended, then refrigerate for about 30 minutes.

4. Cut horizontal pockets into each chicken breast, and stuff them evenly with the filling. Secure the two sides of each breast with toothpicks.

5. Place a large ovenproof skillet over medium-high heat and add the olive oil.

6. Brown the chicken on both sides, about 10 minutes in total.

7. Place the skillet in the oven and roast until the chicken is just cooked through, about 15 minutes. Remove the toothpicks and serve.

Nutrition: Calories: 389 Fat: 30g Protein: 25g Carbohydrates: 3g Fiber: 0g

34. Spicy Pork Chops

Preparation time: 4 hours and 10 minutes

Cooking time: 15 minutes

Servings: 2

Ingredients:

- ¼ cup lime juice 2 pork rib chops
- 1/2 tablespoon coconut oil, melted
- 1/2 garlic cloves, peeled and minced
- 1/2 tablespoon chili powder
- 1/2 teaspoon ground cinnamon
- teaspoon cumin
- Salt and pepper to taste
- 1/4 teaspoon hot pepper sauce
- Mango, sliced

Directions:

1. Take a bowl and mix in lime juice, oil, garlic, cumin, cinnamon, chili powder, salt, pepper, hot pepper sauce. Whisk well.
2. Add pork chops and toss. Keep it on the side, and let it refrigerate for 4 hours.
3. Preheat your grill to medium and transfer pork chops to the preheated grill. Grill for 7 minutes, flip and cook for 7 minutes more.

4. Divide between serving platters and serve with mango slices. Enjoy!

Nutrition: Calories: 200 Fat: 8g Carbohydrates: 3g Protein: 26g Fiber: 1g Net Carbohydrates: 2g

SIDES

35. <u>Simplest Yellow Squash</u>

Preparation Time: 10 minutes

Cooking Time: 12 minutes

Servings: 4

Ingredients:

- 2 tbsp. olive oil
- lb. yellow squash, cut into thin slices
- small yellow onion, cut into thin rings
- garlic clove, minced
- tsp. water
- Salt and freshly ground white pepper, to taste

Directions:

1. In a large skillet, heat the oil over medium-high heat and stir fry the squash, onion and garlic for about 3-4 minutes.
2. Add water, salt and black pepper and stir to combine.
3. Reduce heat to low and simmer for about 6-8 minutes.
4. Serve hot.

Nutrition: Calories: 86; Carbohydrates: 5.7g; Protein: 1.6g; Fat: 7.2g; Sugar: 2.7g; Sodium: 51mg; Fiber: 1.7g

36.   Pumpkin And Cauliflower Rice

Preparation time: 5 minutes

Cooking time: 10 minutes

Servings: 4

Ingredients:

- 2 ounces olive oil
- yellow onion, chopped
- garlic cloves, minced
- 12 ounces cauliflower rice
- cups chicken stock
- 6 ounces pumpkin puree
- ½ teaspoon nutmeg, ground
- teaspoon thyme chopped
- ½ teaspoon ginger, grated
- ½ teaspoon cinnamon powder
- ½ teaspoon allspice
- ounces coconut cream

Directions:

1. Set your instant pot on sauté mode, add the oil, heat it up, add garlic and onion, stir and sauté for 3 minutes.
2. Add cauliflower rice, stock, pumpkin puree, thyme, nutmeg, cinnamon, ginger and allspice, stir, cover and cook on High for 12 minutes.

3. Add coconut cream, stir, divide among plates and serve as a side dish.

4. Enjoy!

Nutrition: Calories 152, fat 2, fiber 3, carbs 5, protein 6

VEGETABLES

37. Fried Eggs with Kale and Bacon

Preparation time: 5 minutes

Cooking time: 15 minutes

Servings: 2

Ingredients:

- 4 slices of turkey bacon, chopped
- bunch of kale, chopped
- oz butter, unsalted
- eggs
- 2 tbsp chopped walnuts
- Seasoning:
- 1/3 tsp salt
- 1/3 tsp ground black pepper

Directions:

1. Take a frying pan, place it over medium heat, add two-third of the butter in it, let it melt, then add kale, switch heat to medium-high level and cook for 4 to 5 minutes until edges have turned golden brown.

2. When done, transfer kale to a plate, set aside until required, add bacon into the pan and cook for 4 minutes until crispy.

3. Return kale into the pan, add nuts, stir until mixed and cook for 2 minutes until thoroughly warmed.

4. Transfer kale into the bowl, add remaining butter into the pan, crack eggs into the pan and fry them for 2 to 3 minutes until cooked to the desired level.

5. Distribute kale between two plates, add fried eggs on the side, sprinkle with salt and black pepper, and then serve.

Nutrition: 525 Calories; 50 g Fats; 14.4 g Protein; 1.1 g Net Carb; 2.8 g Fiber;

38.   <u>Eggs with Greens</u>

Preparation time: 5 minutes

Cooking time: 10 minutes

Servings: 2

Ingredients:

- 3 tbsp chopped parsley
- 3 tbsp chopped cilantro
- ¼ tsp cayenne pepper
- 2 eggs
- tbsp butter, unsalted
- Seasoning:
- ¼ tsp salt
- 1/8 tsp ground black pepper

Directions:

1. Take a medium skillet pan, place it over medium-low heat, add butter and wait until it melts.
2. Then add parsley and cilantro, season with salt and black pepper, stir until mixed and cook for 1 minute.
3. Make two space in the pan, crack an egg into each space, and then sprinkle with cayenne pepper, cover the pan with the lid and cook for 2 to 3 minutes until egg yolks have set.
4. Serve.

Nutrition: 135 Calories; 11.1 g Fats; 7.2 g Protein; 0.2 g Net Carb; 0.5 g Fiber;

39.   Spicy Chaffle with Jalapeno

Preparation time: 5 minutes

Cooking time: 10 minutes;

Servings: 2

Ingredients:

- 2 tsp coconut flour
- ½ tbsp chopped jalapeno pepper
- 2 tsp cream cheese
- egg
- oz shredded mozzarella cheese
- Seasoning:
- ¼ tsp salt
- 1/8 tsp ground black pepper

Directions:

1. Switch on a mini waffle maker and let it preheat for 5 minutes.
2. Meanwhile, take a medium bowl, place all the ingredients in it and then mix by using an immersion blender until smooth.
3. Ladle the batter evenly into the waffle maker, shut with lid, and let it cook for 3 to 4 minutes until firm and golden brown.
4. Serve.

Nutrition: 153 Calories; 10.7 g Fats; 11.1 g Protein; 1 g Net Carb; 1 g Fiber;

40. Pasta Orecchiette with Broccoli & Tofu

Preparation Time: 10 minutes

Cooking Time: 15 minutes

Servings: 4

Ingredients:

- (9 oz.) pack orecchiette
- 16 oz. broccoli, roughly chopped
- garlic cloves
- tbsp. olive oil
- tbsp. grated tofu
- Salt and black pepper to taste

Directions:

1. Place the orecchiette and broccoli in your instant pot. Cover with water and seal the lid. Cook on High Pressure for 10 minutes. Do a quick release.

2. Drain the broccoli and orecchiette. Set aside. Heat the olive oil on Sauté mode. Stir-fry garlic for 2 minutes. Stir in broccoli, orecchiette, salt, and pepper. Cook for 2 more minutes. Press Cancel and Stir in grated tofu, to serve.

Nutrition: Calories: 192 kcal Protein: 7.08 g Fat: 12.6 g Carbohydrates: 16.93 g

SOUPS AND STEWS

41.Pumpkin, Coconut & Sage Soup

Preparation time: 15 minutes

Cooking time: 30 minutes

Servings:6

Ingredients:

- 6 cups vegetable broth

- cup canned pumpkin

- cup full-fat coconut milk

- teaspoon freshly chopped sage

- cloves garlic, chopped

- Pinch of salt & pepper, to taste

Directions:

1. Add all the ingredients minus the coconut milk to a stockpot over medium heat and bring to a boil. Reduce to a simmer and cook for 30 minutes.

2. Add the coconut milk and stir.

Nutrition: Calories: 146 Carbs: 7g Fiber: 2g Net Carbs: 5g Fat: 11g Protein: 6g

42.   Italian Beef Soup

Preparation time: 10 minutes

Cooking time: 4 hours

Servings:6

Ingredients:

- pound lean ground beef
- cup beef broth
- cup heavy cream
- ½ cup shredded mozzarella cheese
- ½ cup diced tomatoes
- 1 yellow onion, chopped
- cloves garlic, chopped
- 1 tablespoon Italian seasoning
- Salt & pepper, to taste

Directions:

1. Add all the ingredients to a slow cooker minus the heavy cream and mozzarella cheese. Cook on high for 4 hours.
2. Warm the heavy cream, and then add the warmed cream and cheese to the soup. Stir well and serve.

Nutrition: Calories: 241 Carbs: 4g Fiber: 1g Net Carbs: 3g Fat: 14g Protein: 25g

DRESSING AND SAUCES

43.   Green Jalapeno Sauce

Preparation Time: 5 minutes

Cooking Time: 0 minutes

Servings: 1

Ingredients:

- ½ avocado

- large jalapeno

- cup fresh cilantro

- tablespoons extra virgin olive oil

- tablespoons water

- Water

- ½ teaspoon salt

Directions:

1. Add all ingredients in a blender.

2. Blend until smooth and creamy.

3. Serve and enjoy.

Nutrition: Calories: 407 Fat: 42g Carbs: 10g Protein: 2.4g

44.   <u>Hot Sauce</u>

Preparation Time: 15 minutes

Cooking Time: 15 minutes

Servings: 40

Ingredients:

- tablespoon olive oil
- cup carrot, peeled and chopped
- ½ cup yellow onion, chopped
- 5 garlic cloves, minced
- 6 habanero peppers, stemmed
- tomato, chopped
- 1 tablespoon fresh lemon zest
- ¼ cup fresh lemon juice
- ¼ cup balsamic vinegar
- ¼ cup water
- Salt and ground black pepper, as required

Directions:

1. Heat the oil in a huge pan over medium heat and cook the carrot, onion, and garlic for about 8-10 minutes, stirring frequently.
2. Remove the pan from heat and let it cool slightly.
3. Place the onion mixture and remaining ingredients in a food processor and pulse until smooth.

4. Return the mixture into the same pan over medium-low heat and simmer for about 3-5 minutes, stirring occasionally.

5. Remove the pan from heat and let it cool completely.

6. You can preserve this sauce in the refrigerator by placing it into an airtight container.

Nutrition: Calories: 9 Net Carbs: 1g Carbohydrate: 1.3g Fiber: 0.3g Protein: 0.2g Fat: 0.4g Sugar: 0.7g Sodium: 7mg

DESSERT

45. Almond Butter Cookies

Preparation Time: 5 minutes

Cooking Time: 12 minutes

Servings: 14

Ingredients:

- 1 cup smooth almond butter
- 4 tbsp unsweetened cocoa powder
- 1/2 cup granulated erythritol sweetener
- 1/4 cup sugar-free chocolate chips
- 1 large egg
- 3 tbsp almond milk unsweetened, if needed

Directions:

1. Preheat your oven at 350 degrees F.
2. Whisk almond butter together with granulated sweetener, egg, and cocoa powder in a bowl with a fork. Add 3 tbsp almond milk if the mixture is too crumbly.
3. Fold in chocolate chips then make 6-centimeterround cookie balls out of it.
4. Place the balls on a baking sheet lined with parchment paper.
5. Bake them for 12 minutes then allow them to cool.
6. Enjoy.

Nutrition: Calories 77.8 Total Fat 7.13 g Total Carbs 0.8 g Sugar 0.2 g Fiber 0.3 g Protein 2.3 g

46.   Macadamia Nut Cookies

Preparation Time: 10 minutes

Cooking Time: 15 minutes

Servings: 12

Ingredients:

- 1/2 cup butter, melted
- 2 tbsp almond butter
- 1 egg
- 1 1/2 cup almond flour
- 2 tbsp unsweetened cocoa powder
- 1/2 cup granulated erythritol sweetener
- 1 tsp vanilla extract
- 1/2 tsp baking soda
- 1/4 cup chopped macadamia nuts
- Pinch of salt

Directions:

1. Preheat your oven to 350 degrees F.
2. Whisk all the ingredients well in a bowl with a fork until smooth.
3. Layer a cookie sheet with wax paper and drop the dough onto it scoop by scoop.
4. Flatten each scoop into 1.5-inch wide round.
5. Bake them for 15 minutes then allow them to cool.

6. Enjoy.

Nutrition: Calories 114 Total Fat 9.6 g Total Carbs 3.1 g Sugar 1.4 g Fiber 1.5 g Protein 3.5 g

47. <u>Cinnamon Roll Muffins</u>

Preparation Time: 5 minutes

Cooking Time: 15 minutes

Servings: 6

Ingredients:

- 1/2 cup almond flour
- 2 scoops vanilla protein powder
- 1 tsp. baking powder
- 1 tbsp. cinnamon
- 1/2 cup almond butter
- 1/2 cup pumpkin puree
- 1/2 cup coconut oil
- For the Glaze
- 1/4 cup coconut butter
- 1/4 cup milk of choice
- 1 tbsp. granulated sweetener
- 2 tsp. lemon juice

Directions:

1. Let your oven preheat at 350 degrees F. Layer a 12-cup muffin tray with muffin liners.
2. Add all the dry ingredients to a suitable mixing bowl then whisk in all the wet ingredients.
3. Mix until well combined then divide the batter into the muffin cups.

4. Bake them for 15 minutes then allow the muffins to cool on a wire rack.

5. Prepare the cinnamon glaze in a small bowl then drizzle this glaze over the muffins.

6. Enjoy.

Nutrition: Calories 252 Total Fat 17.3 g Total Carbs 3.2 g Sugar 0.3 g Fiber 1.4 g Protein 5.2 g

48. Muffins with Blueberries

Preparation Time: 10 minutes

Cooking Time: 25 minutes

Servings: 8

Ingredients:

- 3/4 cup coconut flour
- 6 eggs
- 1/2 cup coconut oil, melted
- 1/3 cup unsweetened coconut milk
- 1/2 cup fresh blueberries
- 1/3 cup granulated sweetener
- 1 tsp. vanilla extract
- 1 tsp. baking powder

Directions:

1. Preheat your oven at 356 degrees F.
2. Mix coconut flour with all the other ingredients except blueberries in a mixing bowl until smooth.
3. Stir in blueberries and mix gently.
4. Divide this batter in a greased muffin tray evenly.
5. Bake the muffins for 25 minutes until golden brown.
6. Enjoy.

Nutrition: Calories 195 Total Fat 14.3 g Total Carbs 4.5 g Sugar 0.5 g Fiber 0.3 g Protein 3.2 g

49.   Chocolate Zucchini Muffins

Preparation Time: 10 minutes

Cooking Time: 30 minutes

Servings: 9

Ingredients:

- 1/2 cup coconut flour
- 3/4 tsp. baking soda
- 2 tbsp. cocoa powder
- 1/2 tsp. salt
- 1 tsp. cinnamon
- 1/2 tsp. nutmeg
- 3 large eggs
- 2/3 cup Swerve sweetener
- 2 tsp. vanilla extract
- 1 tbsp. oil
- 1 medium zucchini, grated
- 1/4 cup heavy cream
- 1/3 cup Lily's chocolate baking chips

Directions:

1. Preheat your oven at 356 degrees F.
2. Layer a 9-cup o muffin tray with muffin liners then spray them with cooking oil.
3. Whisk coconut flour with salt, cinnamon, nutmeg, sweetener, baking soda, and cocoa powder in a bowl.

4. Beat eggs in a separate bowl then add oil, cream, vanilla, and zucchini.

5. Stir in the coconut flour mixture and mix well until fully incorporated.

6. Fold in chocolate chips then divide the batter into the lined muffin cups.

7. Bake these muffins for 30 minutes then allow them to cool on a wire rack.

8. Enjoy.

Nutrition: Calories 151 Total Fat 14.7 g Total Carbs 1.5 g Sugar 0.3 g Fiber 0.1 g Protein 0.8 g

50.   Blackberry-Filled Lemon Muffins

Preparation Time: 5 minutes

Cooking Time: 30 minutes

Servings: 12

Ingredients:

- For the Blackberry Filling:
- 3 tbsp granulated stevia
- 1 tsp lemon juice
- 1/4 tsp xanthan gum
- 2 tbsp water
- 1 cup fresh blackberries
- For the Muffin Batter:
- 2 1/2 cups super fine almond flour
- 3/4 cup granulasted stevia
- 1 tsp fresh lemon zest
- 1/2 tsp sea salt
- 1 tsp grain-free baking powder
- 4 large eggs
- 1/4 cup unsweetened almond milk
- 1/4 cup butter
- 1 tsp vanilla extract
- 1/2 tsp lemon extract

Directions:

1. For the Blackberry Filling:
2. Add granulated sweetener and xanthan gum in a saucepan.

3. Stir in lemon juice and water then place it over the medium heat.

4. Add blackberries and stir cook on low heat for 10 minutes.

5. Remove the saucepan from the heat and allow the mixture to cool.

6. For the Muffin Batter:

7. Preheat your oven at 356 degrees F and layer a muffin tray with paper cups.

8. Mix almond flour with salt, baking powder, lemon zest, baking powder, and sweetener in a mixing bowl.

9. Whisk in eggs, vanilla extract, lemon extract, butter, and almond milk.

10. Beat well until smooth. Divide half of this batter into the muffin tray.

11. Make a depression at the center of each muffin.

12. Add a spoonful of blackberry jam mixture to each depression.

13. Cover the filling with remaining batter on top.

14. Bake the muffins for 30 minutes then allow them to cool.

15. Refrigerate for a few hours before serving.

16. Enjoy.

Nutrition: Calories 261 Total Fat 7.1 g Total Carbs 3.1 g Sugar 2.1 g Fiber 3.9 g Protein 1.8 g

CONCLUSION

Keto can be a great option for people looking to shed extra weight that is stored in their bodies as fat. Ketosis is the process of the body using fats instead of glucose for energy. The liver can take fats and break them down into ketones, which can be used by both the body and the brain as a fuel source. To get the body away from using sugars, however, a person has to severely limit the amount and type of carbs they consume so the body can burn through its glucose stores and start working on the fat stores. This is why it can be so important to stay diligent on the diet once started; otherwise, a person might not see their desired results.

For people who are ready to dedicate themselves 100% to the keto diet, there are various forms of it that can match any person's lifestyle and goals. The standard keto option is best for people trying the diet for the first time because it can be the quickest way to get into ketosis and reap the immediate benefits. There are also cyclical and targeted keto for people who might not be willing to follow the strict diet every day. These options give people an opportunity to consume carbs on certain days based on their own personal plans.

There are many benefits to starting the keto diet beyond just losing weight. Keto can also help people improve their heart health by reducing bad fats and forcing the body to work through fats it has stored, possibly in dangerous places like arteries. It can also help people with certain types of epilepsy reduce seizures by switching the brain onto ketone power. Keto can also help women with PCOS regain their health by promoting weight loss and helping to balance their hormones, which can be a cause of the condition. It can even help clear up acne in some people by reducing blood sugar, which can improve skin conditions.

It is not difficult to switch to and stick to a Keto diet. What is actually difficult is adhering to strict rules and guidelines. As long as you maintain the Fats : Protein : Carbs ratio, you'll lose weight fast. It's a no-brainer. And quite unbecoming that many have deviated from this core principle of the Keto diet. The simple formula is to increase the fat and protein content in your meals and snacks while reducing your carb intake. You must restrict your carb intake to reach and remain in Ketosis. Different people achieve Ketosis with varying amounts of carb intake. Generally, it is easy to reach and stay in Ketosis when you decrease your carb intake to not more than 20grams.

Keeping keto long term can seem difficult for beginners who are just getting used to the mechanics of the diet, but it is not so difficult once they are acclimated to the keto lifestyle. Planning out meals and snacks can help people keep up keto longer because it takes some of the work and thinking out of dieting. A person can simply grab what they need and go. And if the standard keto doesn't work for someone long term, they can refer to the other keto styles to find one that will work for them beyond the initial diet.

Lightning Source UK Ltd.
Milton Keynes UK
UKHW021852010321
379622UK00004B/709